Skylar Learns About Lead Poisoning

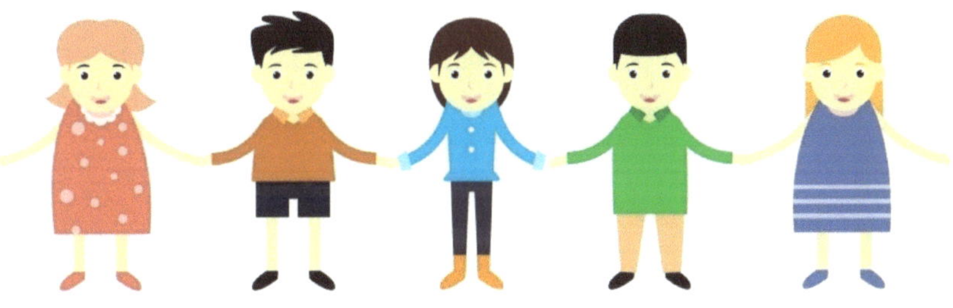

By: Kate Kirkwood

Dedication and Acknowledgement

This book is dedicated to my 4 children, Samantha, Jessyka, Alanna and Skylar, who listened to me read countless hours to them, and inspire me to help protect children around the world from this invisible poison.

Many thanks to my friends and colleagues who encouraged me and helped make this book possible Mark Jacobsen, Tamara Rubin, Ralph Reigh Degoma, Gloria Paradise, Beverly Drouin, and Lisa Parda.

Edited by Scarlett Savage

Published by North East Health & Housing

ISBN-13: 978-1985884991
ISBN-10: 1985884992

"Hi honey, how was school today?" asked Skylar's mom, smiling. It was a favorite part of the day for them both when they talked about everything Skylar had learned in school that day.

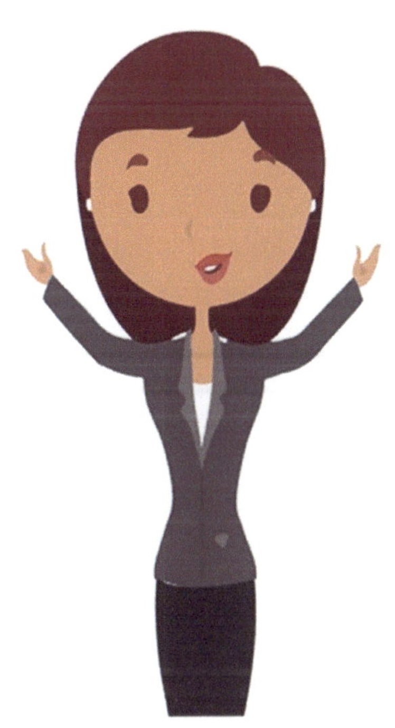

"Good," Skylar told her. "Nurses came to the school to teach us some things."

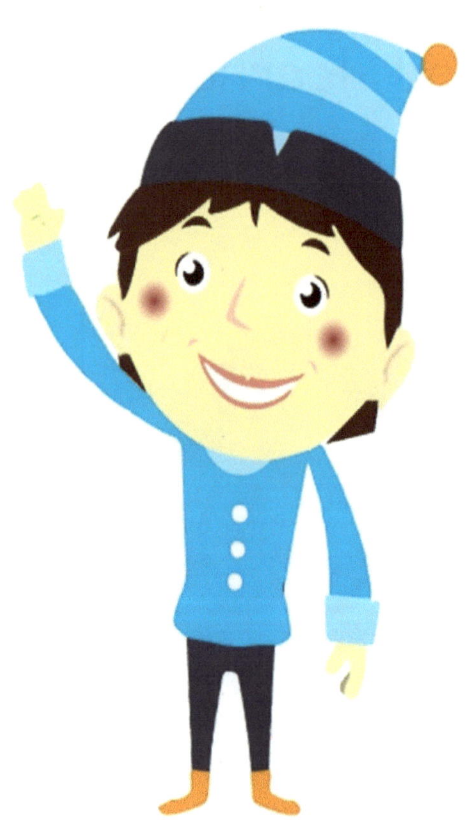

4

Oh? What did nurses teach you?" asked Skylar's Mom, pulling open the refrigerator door--which was covered with Skylar's artwork, and pouring them both a glass of juice.

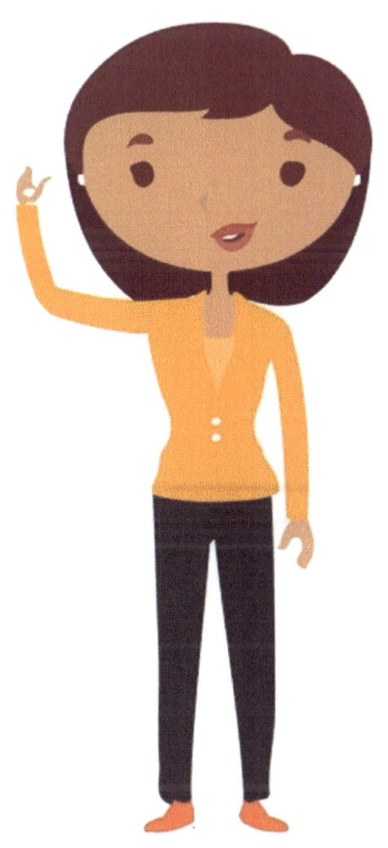

"About lead poisoning," Skylar told her, "and that it can make you very, very sick."

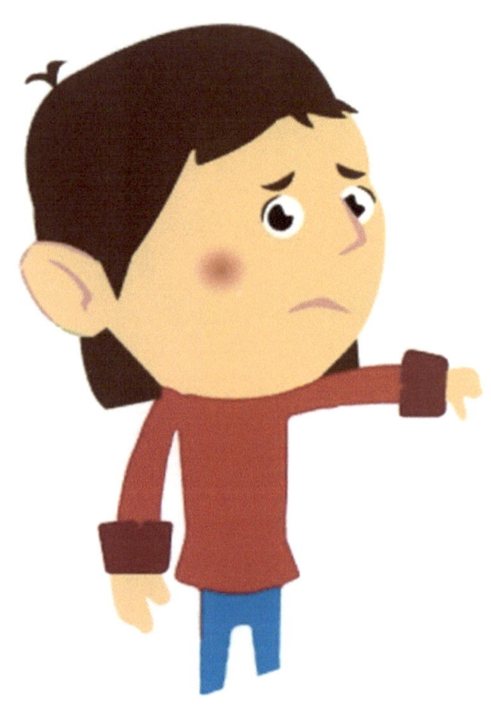

"You know, that's exactly right," Skylar's Mom agreed. smiling. She was proud of how Skylar loved to learn new things. "It can come from lots of places, from old toys, and from the paint in old houses, too."

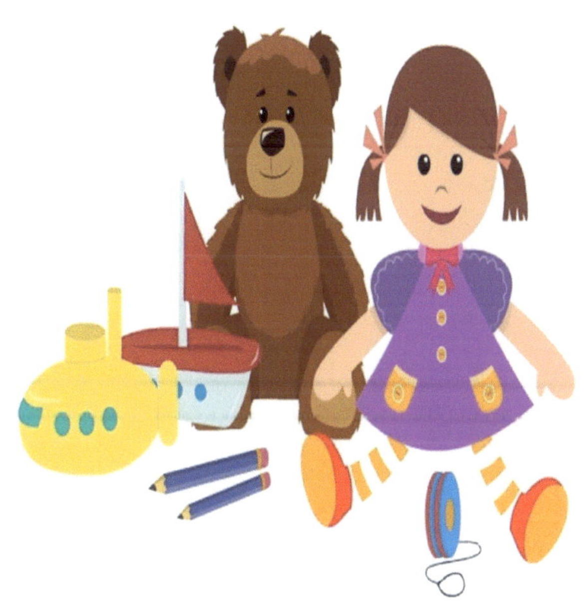

"First, we played a guessing game with some pictures, Mom, and I can show you," Skylar took some pictures out of a backpack. "See? The teacher gave us these five pictures, and we had to guess which ones had lead, and the ones that had lead could make us sick."

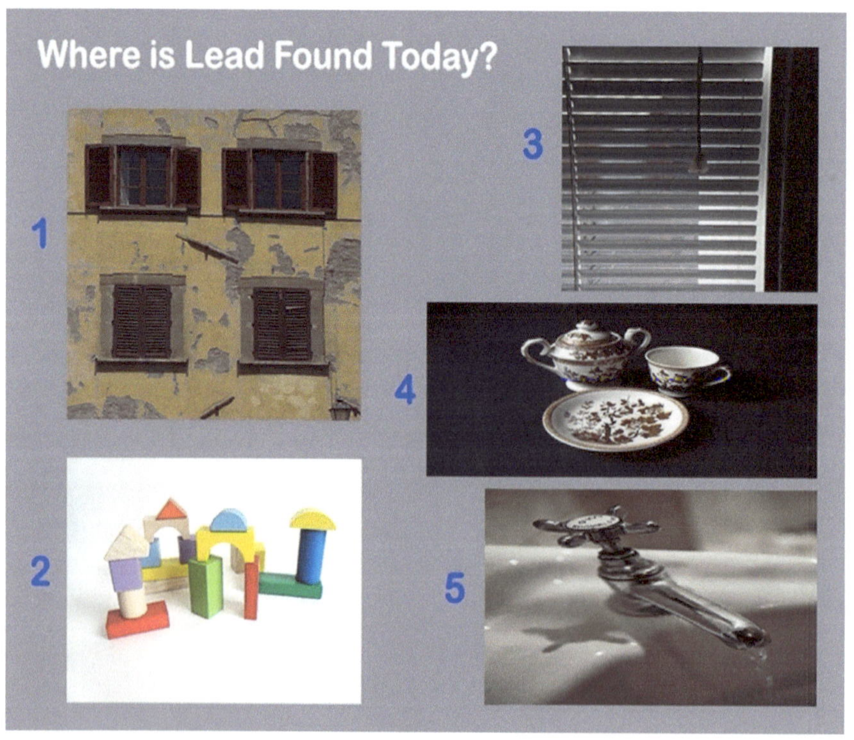

Skylar's Mom was very interested now. "Well, let's play!"

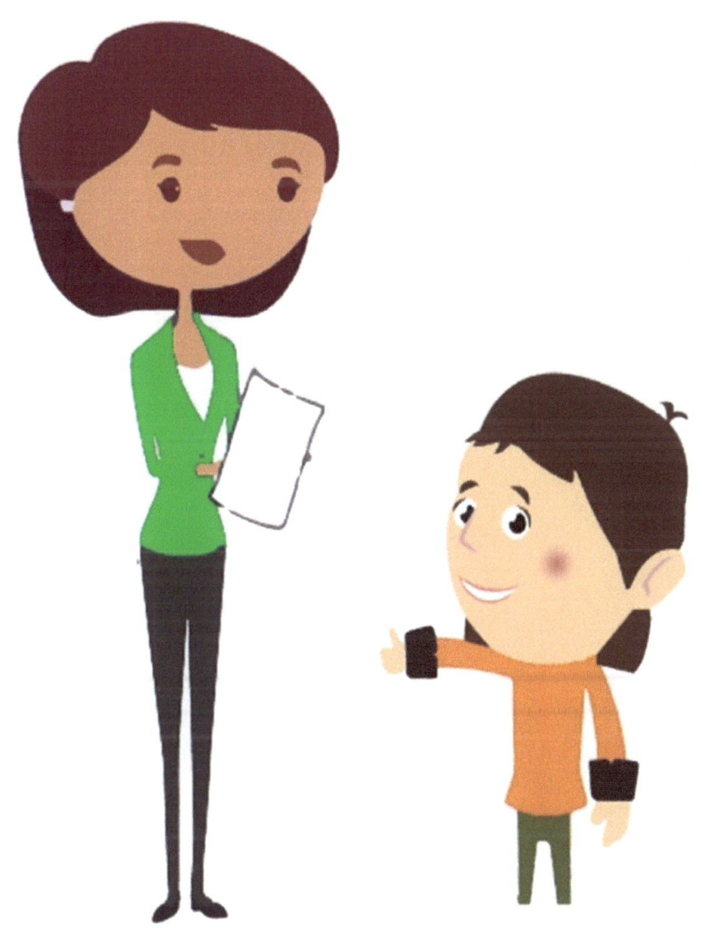

"Here's the first picture," Skylar
showed her. "What do you think?"

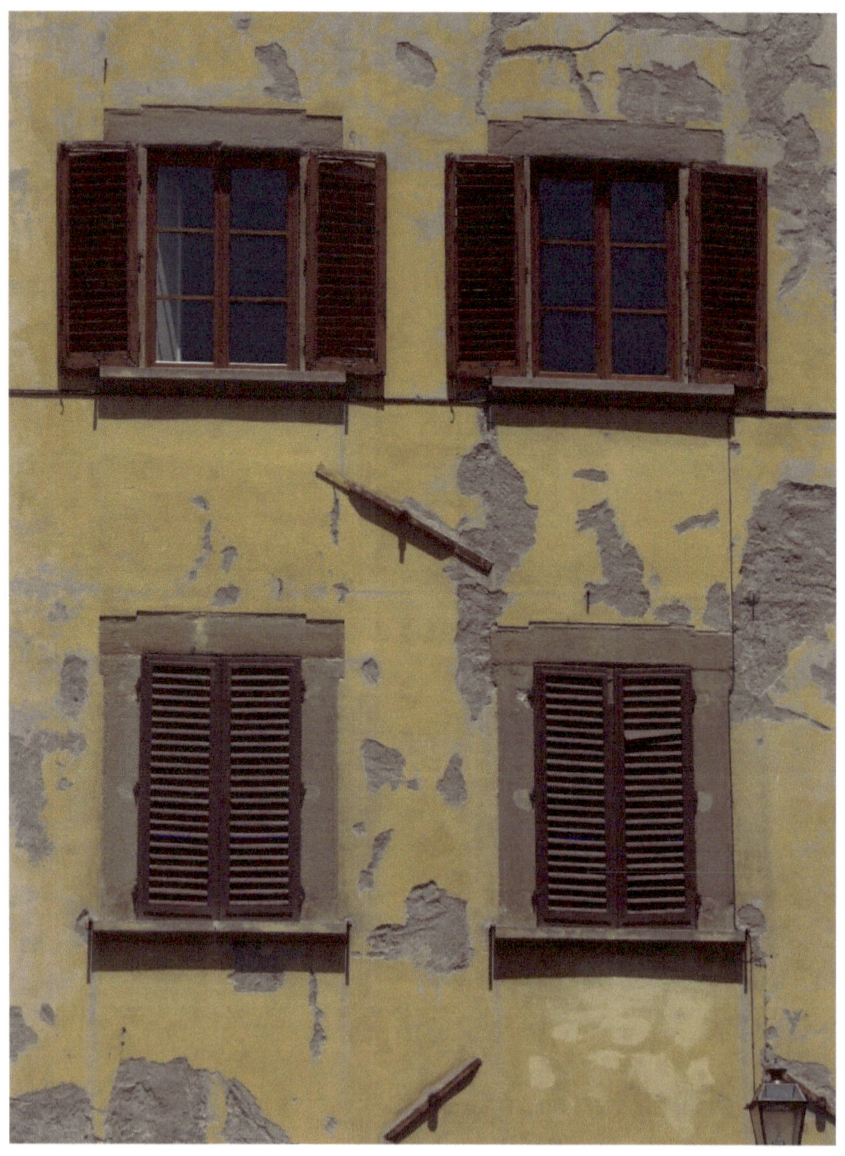

"That's an easy one," Mom pointed out, "because it's an old house, and it's covered in old paint. A lot of old paint had lead in it--"

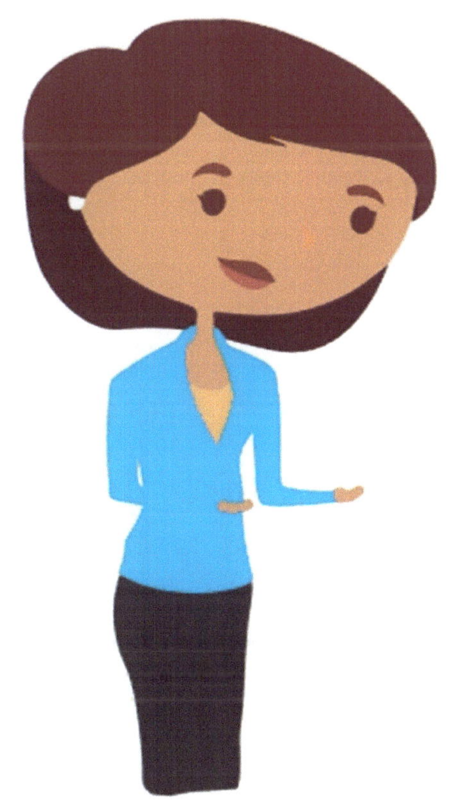

Why?" Skylar blurted out quickly, and then said "Ooops! I know I'm not supposed to interrupt, Mom, I just got excited"

Mom smiled knowingly. She was proud of Skylar's enthusiasm about learning something new.

"People put lead in the paint because it made it last longer, and it was stronger paint. They used lead in a lot of things we'd never use it in today--did you know that the first Queen Elizabeth used makeup that had lead in it?"

Skylar's jaw dropped. "No way!"

"Oh, yes, indeed!" said Mom.

"Anyway, back to the picture...you should always be careful of paint, but especially old paint that is chipping and peeling,"

It was fun to hear about people from long ago, but it's a good thing mom doesn't wear makeup with lead in it today. Skylar thought.

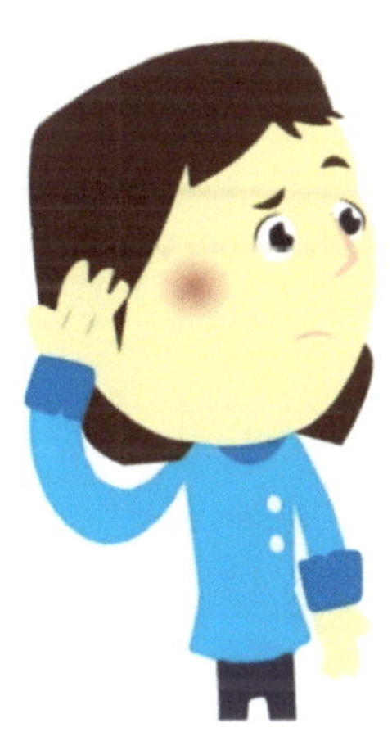

13

"Here's picture number two,"
Skylar said out loud "It's toys,
and you just said that old toys
often have lead paint on them,
right?"

"Yes, dear, that's right!" Mom
smiled again. "Good listening!!!
Parents have to be very careful,
and have the toys tested, and be
sure that there's no chipping or
peeling paint."

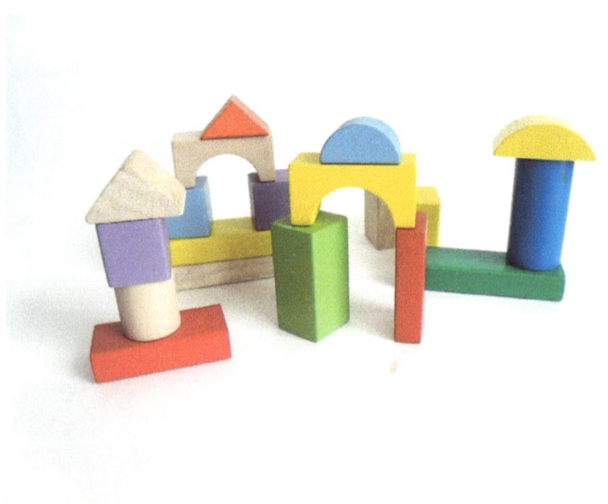

"Here's picture number three,"
Skylar took up the next picture.
"This is an easy one, because it's
window blinds--no lead there."

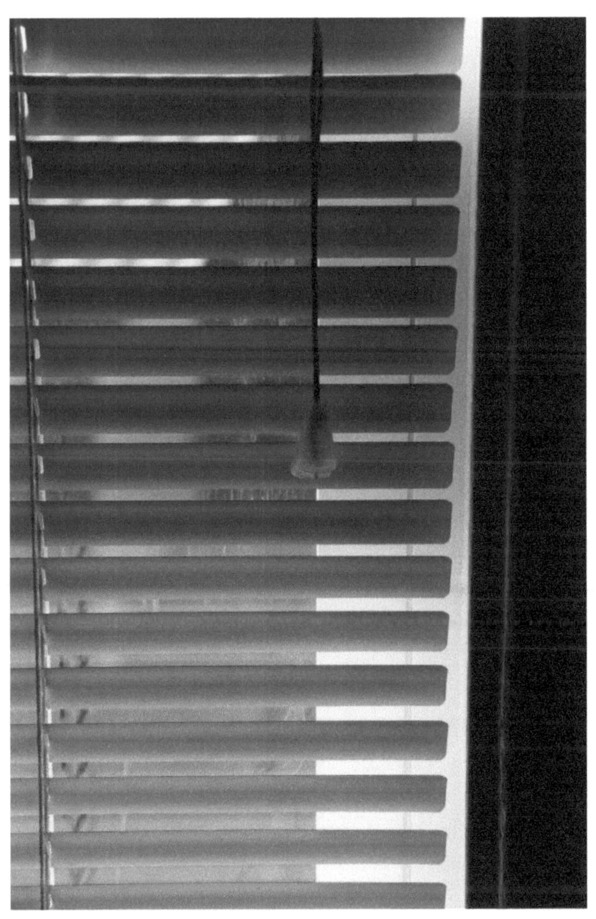

"Actually, there's no paint, but there still could be lead," Mom explained.

"Really?" Skylar asked, with a wrinkled nose "But...how?"

"Because sometimes these kinds of blinds are packaged in a fine layer of dust...and sometimes there are tiny pieces of lead in the dust, or in the plastic itself."

"There can be lead in dust?" Skylar couldn't believe it. This was certainly a very strange but interesting conversation.

Mom nodded.

"That's why I'm always reading the packaging very, very carefully to make sure that I don't accidentally buy something that has lead in it."

"So that's why!" Skylar had teased her before when she'd seemed to take a long time in the stores as she read the labels. "Now I know why you are a slow shopper!"

Mom sighed
"Yes, my dear, that's why."

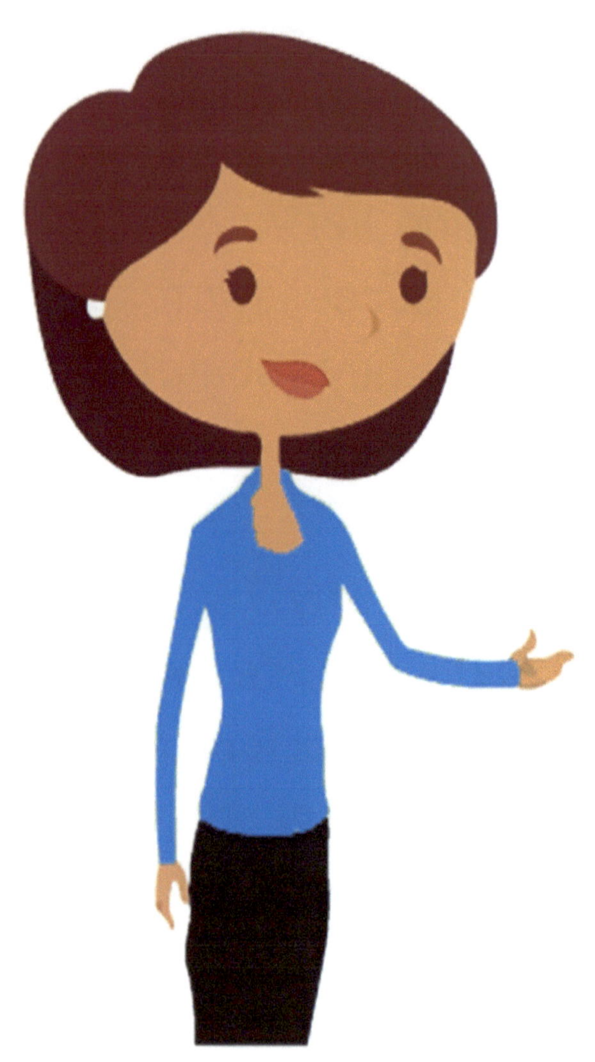

"On to picture number four, Now, don't try to trick me, because there's sure no way that there's lead in dishes, Mom."

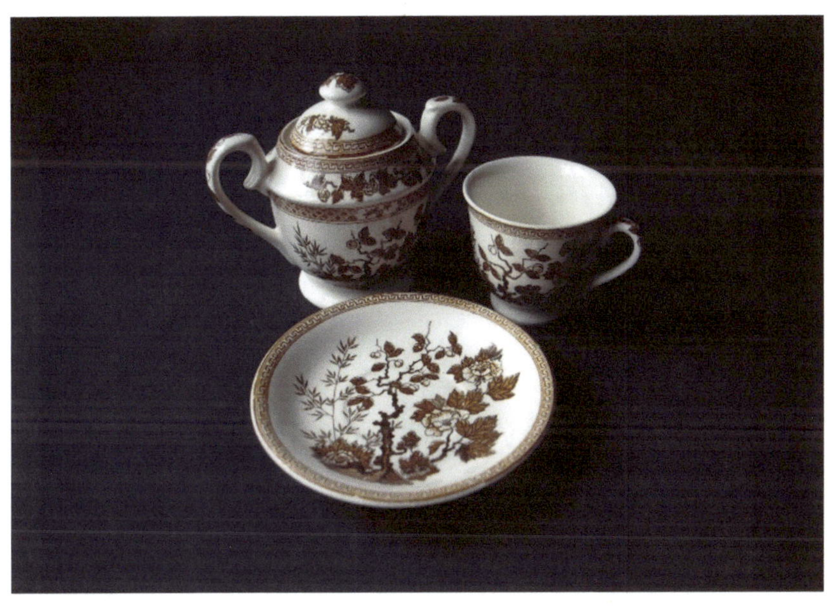

"Actually," Skylar's Mom was already reading the information. "It says here that some pottery and glass contain lead."

"So we have to make sure to ask before we buy them?"

"Yes--that, or we can actually test it ourselves with a little kit that we can buy at the store."

"Really? Where?"

"Apparently the EPA has recognized two kits, Lead-Check and D-Lead that are inexpensive and available on-line and in some paint and hardware stores. If we follow the directions carefully these kits will tell us if the dishes have lead or not"

"Wow, can we get some?" Skylar asked.

"You bet!" and she added a note to the shopping list on the fridge.

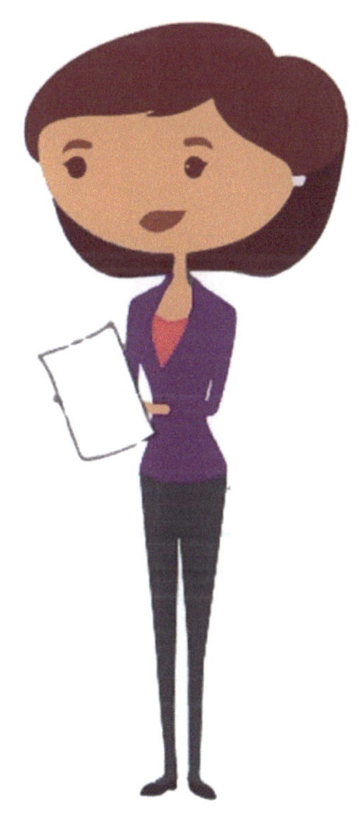

21

And last of all, picture number five shows that even water sometimes contains lead, because sometimes the pipes that carry the water are made of lead. But, it's very easy to test water, to make sure it's safe." Skylar ended with a flourish.

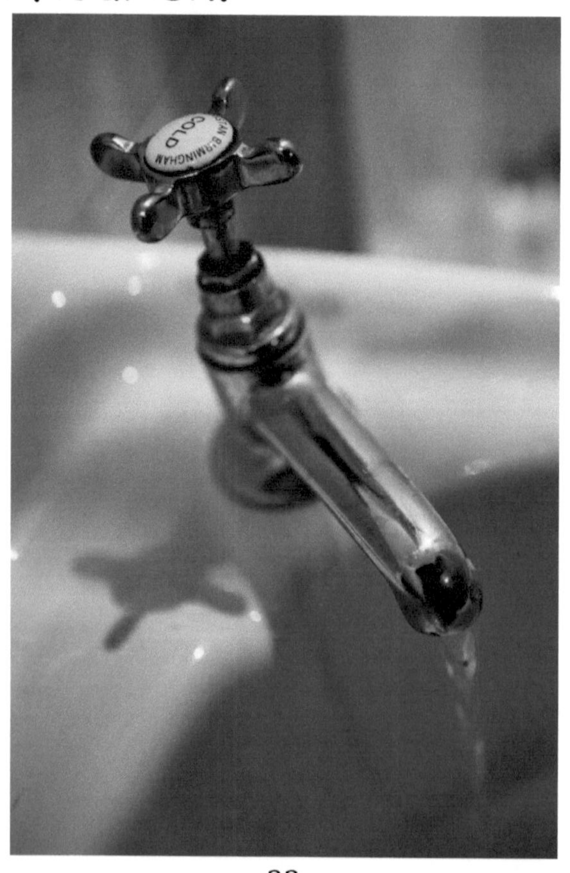

"And, if we are worried about it, it's always a good idea to use a water filter to make sure any bad things that are in the water are filtered out." Added Mom

"Like the cool water pitcher that your friend Scarlett got you for a present last year?" Skylar asked, referring to one of his mom's closest friends.

"Yes—the research isn't clear about filters and lead in the water, but I think it can't hurt since we drink a lot of water to stay healthy, so we use a filter to help keep us safe."

"Plus, it tastes WAY better," Skylar pointed out. Skylar's mom couldn't disagree with that--she used the pitcher Scarlett had given her all the time.

Skylar put the pictures away, suddenly feeling a bit uneasy.

"You know, Mom, I don't think I like this game....there are so many places we can get exposed to lead--it's really scary, Mom"

Sky played with the empty juice glass - "I don't want to get sick."

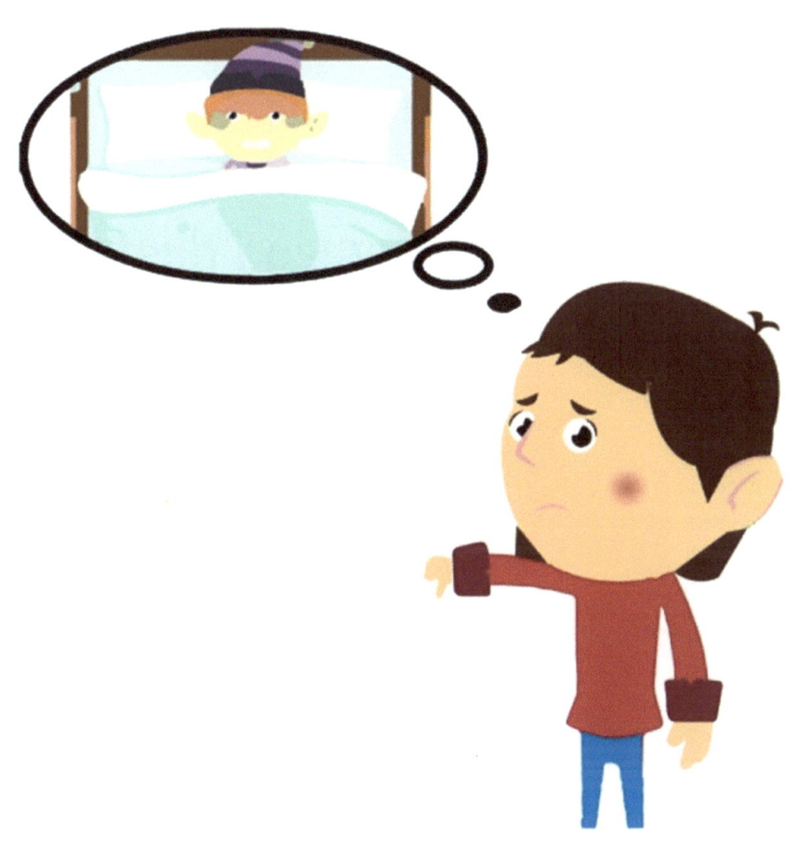

"Don't worry, sweetheart,"
assured Mom, "you won't get
sick...as long as you're careful.

That's why the nurses came to your school today, to teach you how to make sure that you do not eat or breath in any lead dust."

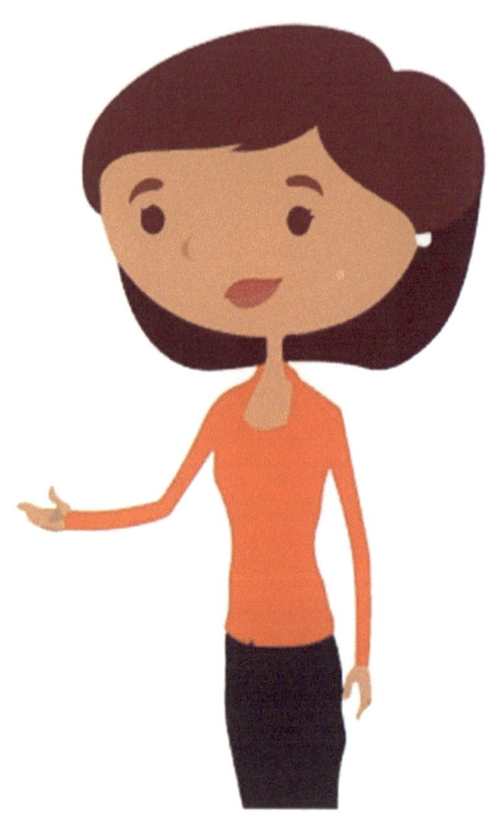

"How else can I be careful?"
Skylar wanted to know.

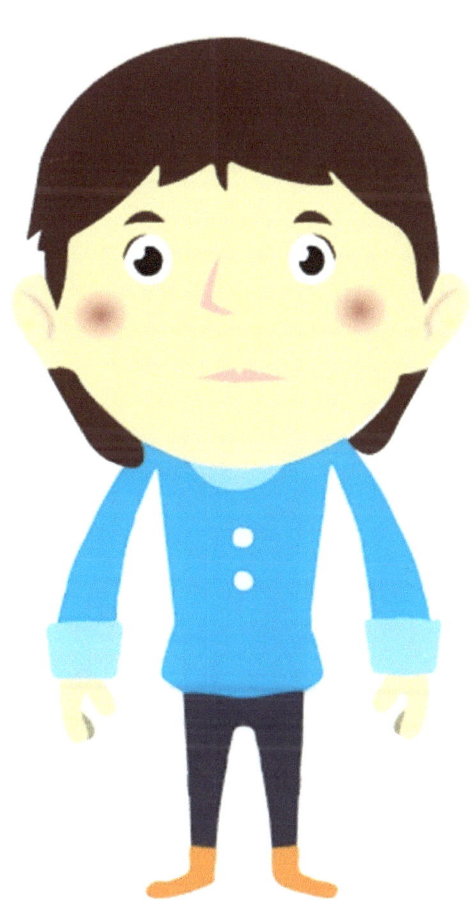

"Well, first we must always remember to wash our hands after playing outside in the dirt." said Mom.

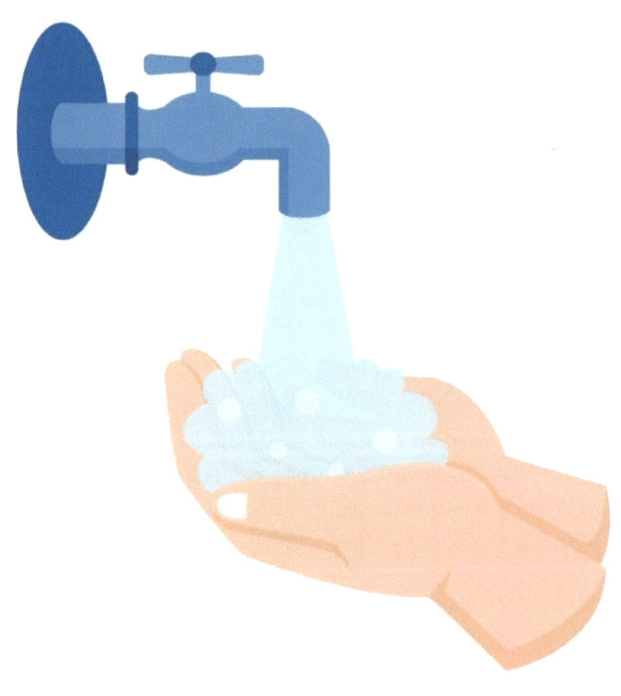

"That's what the nurse said too. And before we eat, right Mom?" said Skylar.

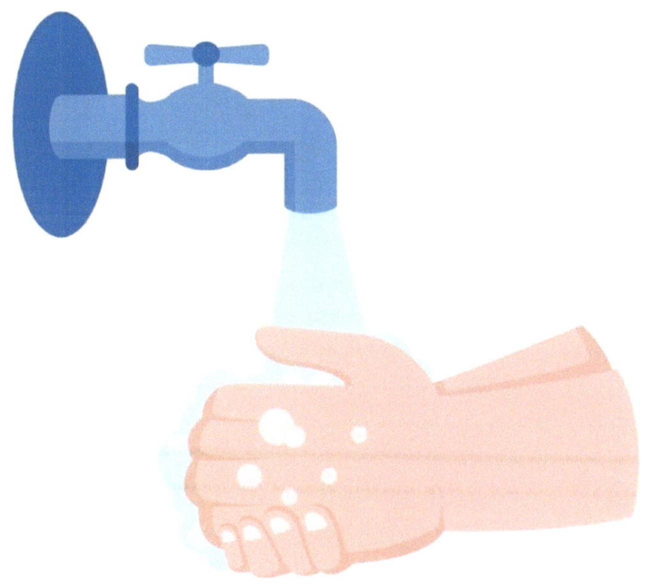

"Yes, before you eat every single meal, even if it's just a snack," Skylar's Mom agreed. "We can help each other remember that--you know I forget that one sometimes, too."

"When else should we wash our hands?" Skylar wanted to know. "I really, REALLY hate getting sick!"

Skylar's Mom thought about it for a moment. "After bathroom and outside time, Before bedtime, before naptime.

And," she emphasized, "We must remember it's never a good idea to put your hands or your toys in your mouth, ever."

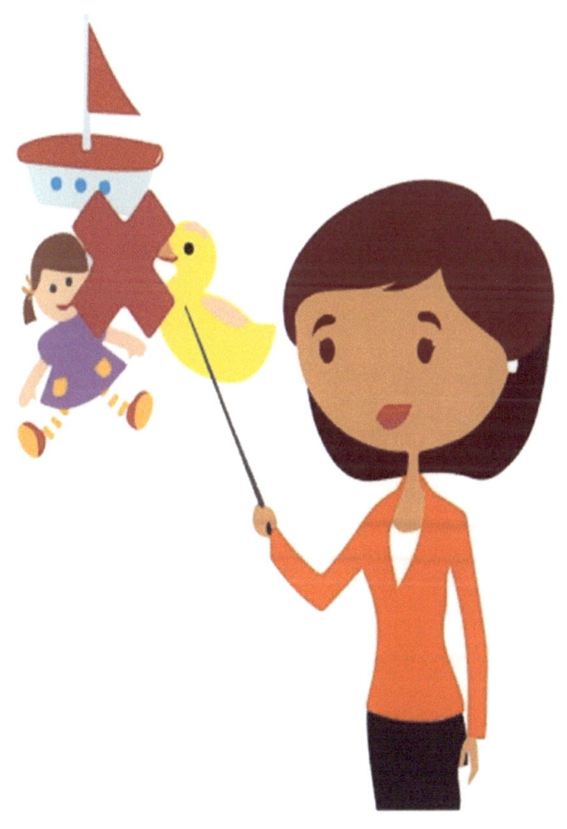

Skylar suddenly remembered something else. "The nurses also said that sometimes, parents have certain jobs, and they can accidentally bring home lead dust with them. Is that true?"

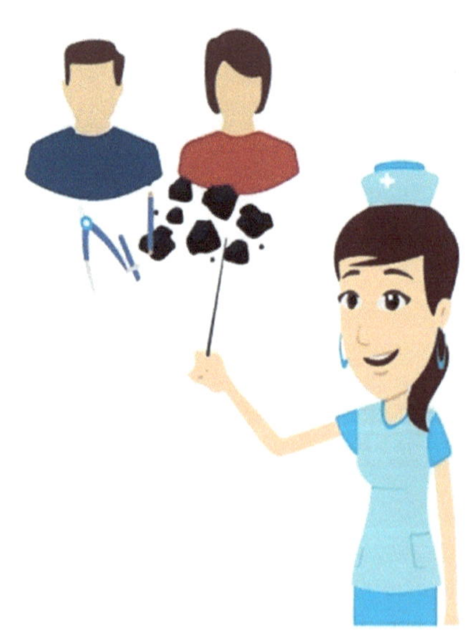

"It sure is," his Mom told him.

"Your daddy, fixes old houses, so he not only washes his hands, but changes his clothes into home clothes before he even comes in to give you a hug."

"Really? Why?" Skylar asked. "I didn't know daddy did that."

"Remember we talked about how there can be lead dust in old houses, or lead paint?" she asked, and Skylar nodded.

"Well, when he works on those houses, sometimes invisible bits of lead dust can get onto his clothes and shoes."

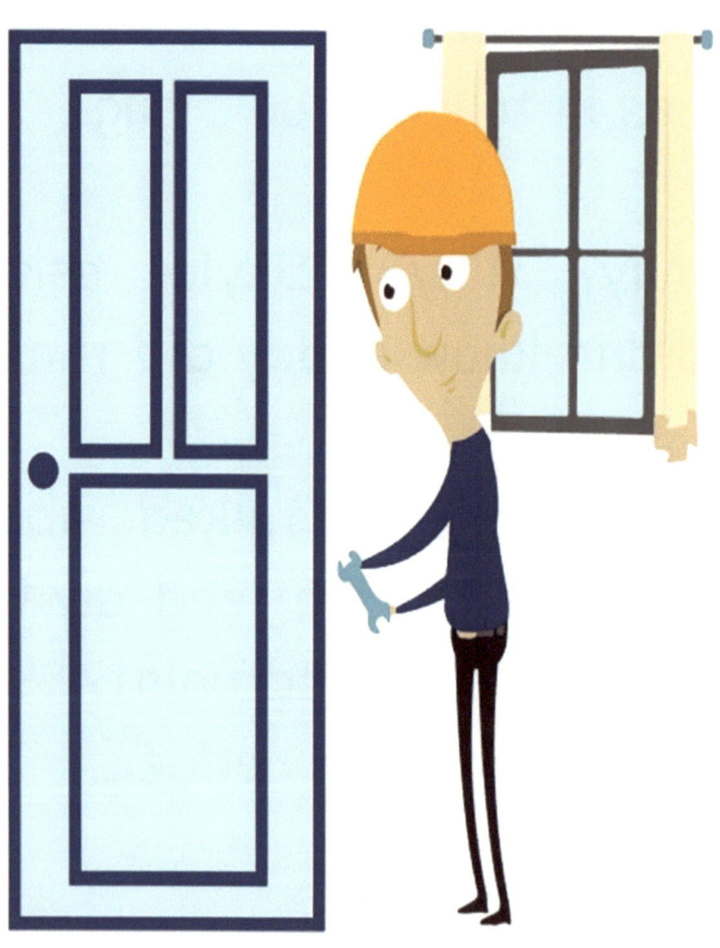

Skylar suddenly remembered something.

"Mom, look! The nurses gave me this paper to show you."

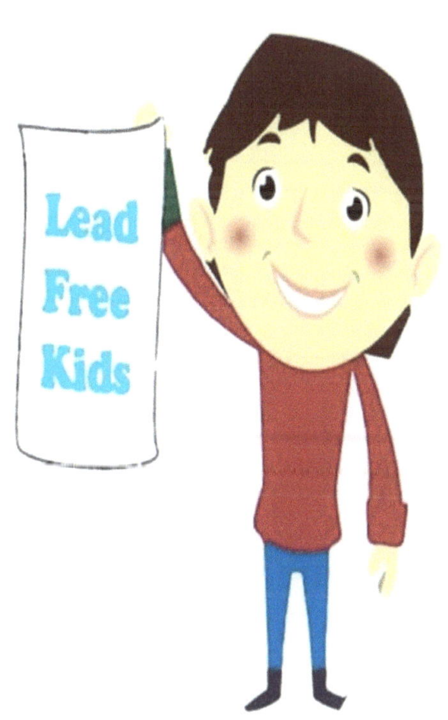

"Oh, great!" Mom was delighted. "It's a flyer for free lead testing for all the kids in our town."

"Did I ever get one, Mom?" asked Skylar.

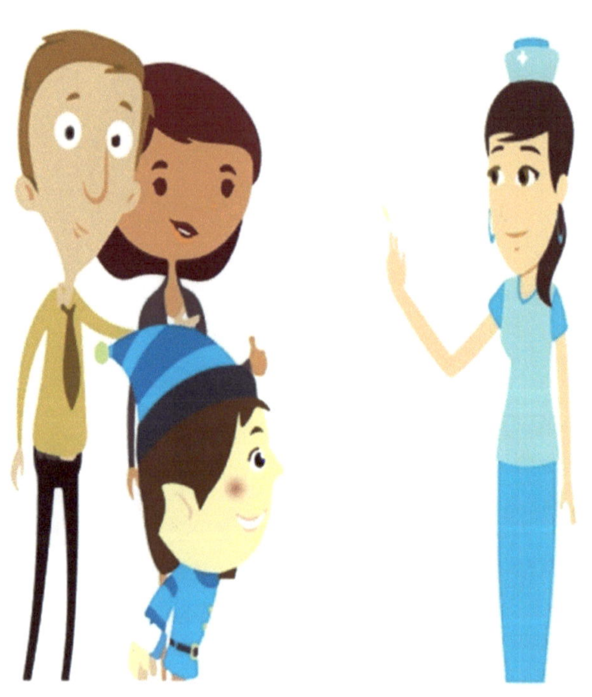

You sure did, honey--in fact, all children should get a lead test at ages one and two. You got both tests, and you were perfectly fine."

"What about James?" Skylar asked anxiously.

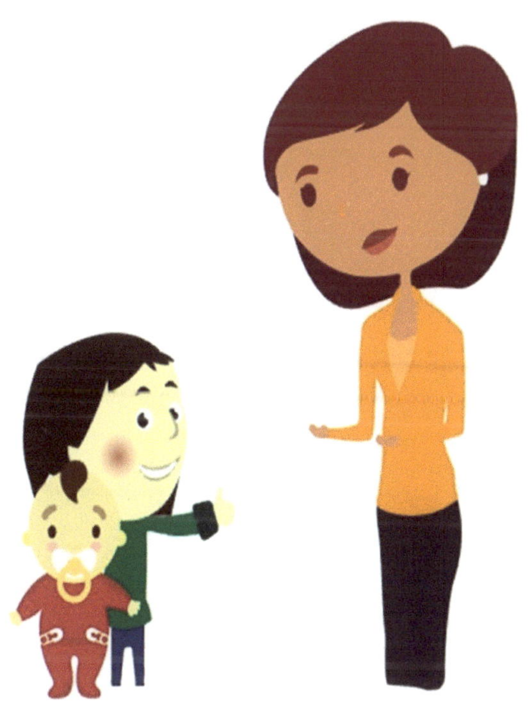

"Your little brother needs to be tested, especially since we moved into this house, which was built before 1978--that's when they began making sure that they didn't use lead paint any more in houses, So, we'll take him to see the public health nurse."

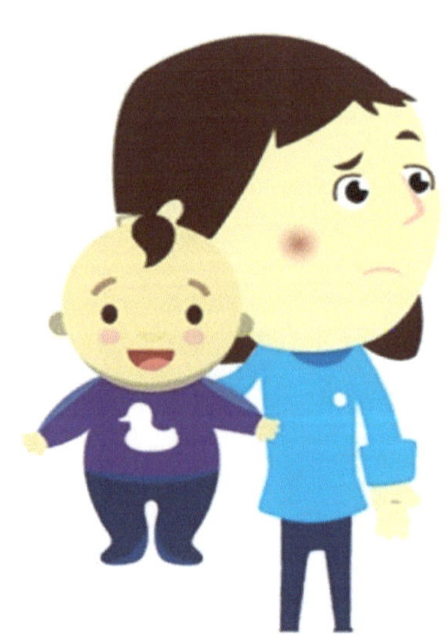

"Good," Skylar was relieved.

"Mom, can I tell you something?"

"Of course, sweetheart. What is it?"

Skylar took a deep breath, thinking. "This was a scary conversation...because of all the things that have lead in them, that I didn't know about. But, now that the nurses taught us some things, and you explained all this stuff to me, I know how to be careful.

Now that you answered all my questions, and I know how to be safe, I feel much better. So, thank you."

"You're welcome, honey," Skylar's Mom smiled. "That's why it's so important, when you have questions, especially about your health--that you bring them up to your parents, or the school nurse, and get answers.

I always say....
Information keeps you safe."

"Information keeps you safe!"
Skylar repeated. "That's my
new favorite saying!"
Mom laughed. "Then let's say it
together, loud and proud, one,
two, three!!"

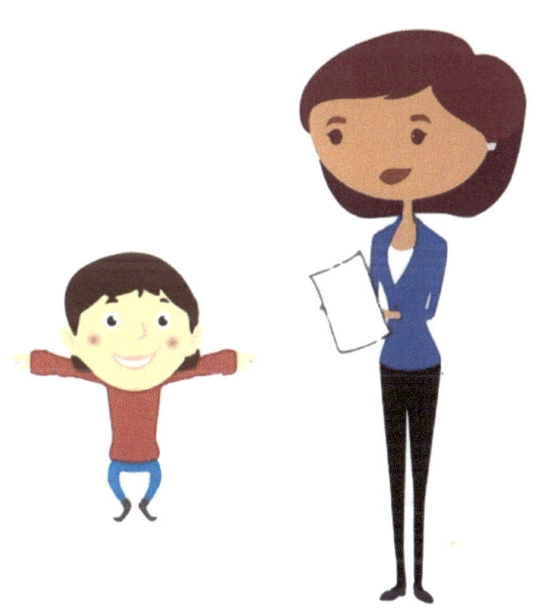

INFORMATION KEEPS YOU SAFE!!

In this story, Mom and Skylar keep changing clothes to show that this can be any Mom, and Skylar can be any girl or boy, in any house, on any day.

Please get your child tested for lead if you have not already done so.

Lead screenings are offered through your local health department, Doctor's office, hospital or WIC Clinic.

Contact them as soon as possible.

For more information visit
www.leadpaintclearandsimple.com

or contact
Kate Kirkwood
603-781-4304
kate@leadpaintclearandsimple.com

Published by

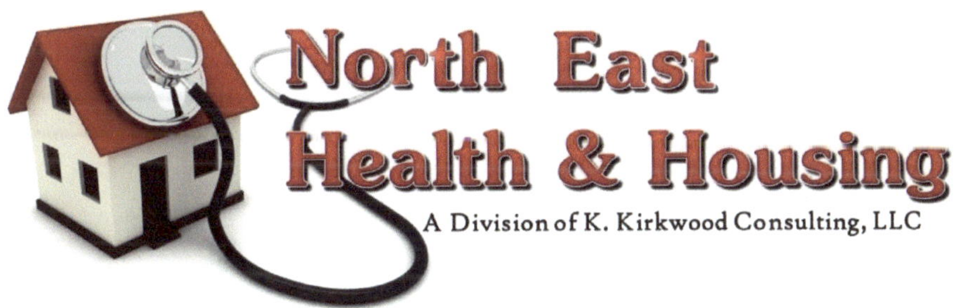